clean body

the humble art of zen-cleansing yourself

by michael dejong

a joost elffers production

STERLING

New York / London
www.sterlingpublishing.com

STERLING and the distinctive Sterling logo are registered trademarks of
Sterling Publishing Co., Inc.

10 9 8 7 6 5 4 3 2 1

Published by Sterling Publishing Co., Inc.
387 Park Avenue South, New York, NY 10016

This book is printed in a sustainable manner using 100 percent (post- and pre-consumer) recycled
paper and vegetable-based inks. No new trees were used.

Copyright © 2009 by Michael DeJong and Joost Elffers Books

CLEAN BODY
The Humble Art of Zen-Cleansing Yourself
A Joost Elffers Production

Distributed in Canada by Sterling Publishing
c/o Canadian Manda Group, 165 Dufferin Street
Toronto, Ontario, Canada M6K 3H6
Distributed in the United Kingdom by GMC Distribution Services
Castle Place, 166 High Street, Lewes, East Sussex, England BN7 1XU
Distributed in Australia by Capricorn Link (Australia) Pty. Ltd.
P.O. Box 704, Windsor, NSW 2756, Australia

Design and illustration by Yumi Asai and Edgar Prieto at Berrymatch LLC

Printed in China
All rights reserved

Sterling ISBN 978-1-4027-6679-4

For information about custom editions, special sales, premium and
corporate purchases, please contact Sterling Special Sales
Department at 800-805-5489 or specialsales@sterlingpublishing.com.

....

I'm clean because of the support
of those around me.

Acknowledgments

To Mrs. Hoogeveen, my childhood neighbor and babysitter, to my maternal Dutch-born grandma, *and* to my mom—who all scrubbed me so hard I appeared sunburned even in the winter.

To my barber who, one day, surprisingly shaved my balding head and promised I'd thank him later. Thank you!

To our over-groomed dog, Jack, because he patiently lets me bathe him. Wash, rinse, and repeat. Wash, rinse, and repeat. Wash, rinse, and repeat.

To Joost Elffers because he understands the way I vibrate.

And to my Richard, just "so-cause."

Index

8

	baking soda	lemon	olive oil	salt	white vinegar	pages
Citrus derma-dip		x	x	x		134
Citrus quaff-conditioner		x				75
Corn removal		x				66
Cuticle conditioner			x			87
D						
Dandruff treatment		x				121
Deep-conditioning						
hair/scalp treatment			x			124
Denture cleaner					x	94
Discolored elbows		x				47
Discolored knees		x				47
Dry shampoo	x					74
E						
Elbow callus remover		x				46 • 47
Elbow deep cleaning	x					45
Elbow exfoliate				x		46

	baking soda	lemon	olive oil	salt	white vinegar	pages
F						
Facial acne					x	55
Facial antiseptic				x		53
Facial astringent		x				55
Facial disinfectant				x		54
Facial exfoliate				x		54
Facial moisturizer			x			56
Facial scrub	x					53
Facial toner					x	56
Foot deodorant	x					64
Foot massage		x	x			68
Foot moisturizer			x			67
Foot soak	x					64
Foot tonic				x	x	68
H						
Hair clarifying paste	x					73
Hair highlights		x				75
Hair-product residue removal					x	76

	baking soda	lemon	olive oil	salt	white vinegar	pages
Hand cleaner	x					82
Hand deodorizer					x	86
Hand exfoliation			x	x		84
Hand moisturizer			x			86
Hand soak	x					83
Hand softener		x				84
I						
Itchy booty					x	142
Itchy scalp		x				121
Itchy skin relief		x				105 • 131
K						
Kinky hair			x			78
Knee callus remover		x				46 • 47
Knee deep cleaning	x					45
Knee exfoliate				x		46

	baking soda	lemon	olive oil	salt	white vinegar	pages
L						
Lice			x			122
M						
Makeup remover			x			58
Moisturizing facial scrub			x	x		58
Moisturizing hair treatment			x			76
Moisturizing hand treatment		x	x			88
Mouthwash	x					91
N						
Nail hardener			x			87
O						
Oily face					x	56
Oral rinse				x		93
P						
Pesky dandruff					x	122

	baking soda	lemon	olive oil	salt	white vinegar	pages
Sunburn					×	132
T						
Toothpaste	×					91
V						
Vaginal cleanser					×	106
W						
Whitehead treatment				×		54
Z						
Zit-zapper				×		54

Preface

Okay, I admit it—I'm a clean freak. In fact, I'm proud of it!

I clean stuff, sometimes twice—the dishes, pots, pans, floors, rugs, windows, bedding, our poor dog Jack, and myself. I also clean right behind my partner, Richard, which drives him totally nuts. I know it's annoying, but nothing ever seems clean enough. And I just can't help it—it's in my genes. Like Joan Crawford in *Mommy Dearest*, "It's the dirt I hate!"

I am a wiper, too. You know, one of those people who always has a sink full of bubbles and a clean wet rag at the ready, just in case.

When I moved to New York in 1987 to be an artist, I was already aware of my "special" needs. Some might call them obsessions, but I prefer to call them standards. I like a clean home and orderly storage. I want my junk where I can find it, and I want it all to look like something. So when I worked as a housekeeper, it not only offered me a vehicle for the overflow of inexhaustible cleaning energy, it also gave me license to police the homes of others as well. It was nothing for me to rearrange my clients'

entire rooms—something that was usually greatly appreciated...
though sometimes not.

I clean with abandon and the effects are swell: shiny floors, spot-
less counters, sparkly refrigerator interiors, crisp white sheets,
and a dust-and-dander-free environment to the best of my
ability. Our friends, Anne and Angi, jokingly refer to our house as
"The Museum," yet our house is very much lived in—we actually
eat, entertain, play, and work in every room of our home. But I
like to leave a room the way I found it—clean and tidy. And, as
much as I am able, the cleaning happens almost entirely with the
use of homemade cleansers Richard and I make from scratch.

Strong and tall as I am, deep down I'm ultra-sensitive to my
surrounding environment. These days, everything makes me
sneeze. Watery eyes, a stuffy nose, and irritated skin are a continual burden. Not just commercial cleaning products, but most
grooming aids and anything with a perfumed scent, leave me
choking. Gourmet soaps, yummy gels, scented moisturizers,
deodorants, and sometimes even shaving cream make me
aggravated, sensitive, and flaky (okay... *flaky-er*).

I needed a solution to all these harsh chemicals and artificial scents, and this is how I came by it. I began to realize that the beauty products we take for granted as a part of modern life didn't always exist. The lotions and potions that come from behind glass counters packaged in tiny jars, tubes, and pumps are actually relatively new—most were only introduced in the last half of the twentieth century. Pilgrims traveled, pirates pillaged, cowboys rustled, prairie women homesteaded, and explorers sailed from one flat edge of the planet to the other without any need for cuticle cream, pop-up wipes, or volumizing shampoo-and-conditioner-in-one treatments. And even despite the lack of indoor plumbing, most found adequate ways to keep clean—well, once they realized that bathing was actually good for them.

Today, I use almost nothing at all that I don't make myself, and I have gone for years and years using limited (and mostly hypoallergenic) commercial products. Although I may never make *People* magazine's "50 Most Beautiful" list, and despite my aversion to the aforementioned goos, gels, and grooming aids, I pride myself on my healthy skin.

Don't get me wrong—there are many fine commercial products on the market that work well and are in harmony with the environment. So if you have found some that agree with you, by all means, stick with them. But at the same time, as mindful Zen-Cleansers, we all need to think about the eco-unfriendly stuff that is being foisted upon us on TV, in magazines, and on the Internet. Until we know what we are wiping, daubing, smearing, or spreading all over ourselves, these *Clean Body* tried-and-true, safe-and-sound "green" potions might just be the best for our bodies, our families, and our planet.

INTRODUCTION

"All the beauty of the world, 'tis but skin deep."
~RALPH VENNING

"Keep yourself pure..."
~THE BOOK OF TIMOTHY

Don't know about you, but I love to lie in the bathtub. I can sometimes soak for hours. It's something I've done my whole life. One of my greatest guilty pleasures is to spend an entire afternoon behind a closed door, unscented candles burning, listening to National Public Radio or music on our tinny waterproof radio, often paging through shiny magazines and luxuriating in the hot swirling water while billows of steam coat and moisten every inch of the room. It makes me relax and unwind to the point that I sometimes even nap while immersed—*not* recommended, by the way!

When I've finished soaking, I'll shower off and then can spend as much time out of the tub grooming as I did steeping in the bath itself.

The importance of cleanliness and good personal hygiene is something that was taught to me and my siblings from very early on. Ingrained in us were notions that we should be "pure," which we, as children, understood to mean "clean and fresh." But for active kids like us, growing up in the suburbs of Chicago, that was no small feat. It meant scrubbing our hands, teeth, hair, and skin, getting the glop out from under our nails and the gum from our hair, and scraping the mountains of dirt from our ears. It meant scrubbing so hard with the washcloth that our skin turned red. Our mom mandated cleaning as an exercise meant not only to bring us self-esteem, but also to spread happiness to those around us: "Oh, that Ruth DeJong—she has the most spick-and-span kids in the neighborhood!" Of course, beneath the skin-deep surface of cleanliness was an implied freshness of spirit and soul; we had also metaphorically washed away the "sins" of the day.

Other than my indulgent tub soaks, I'm not that different from anyone else. As an average American adult, I bathe every day, floss not nearly as often as I should, and brush my teeth far too vigorously. I scrub and pumice, tweeze and trim, wash, swab, polish, and rinse. As the bottle suggests, I sometimes even repeat.

When it comes to personal hygiene, culturally, we are an obsessive lot. We grab just about any grooming product that promises to magically do the job: milky moisturizers, gooey masks, scented shampoos, slippery scrubs, silky powders, youth-enhancing wrinkle creams, and rich, luxurious gels. But truth-be-told, most of the contents in our favorite products are untested and unregulated. "Why worry?" you might ask. "It's about time we started worrying!" say I. When I recently learned that 89 percent of all cosmetic products have *not* undergone safety testing, I freaked. No wonder I blister when I use some products, break out when I'm subjected to others, and have sneezing fits when exposed to yet others. I'd fallen victim to the hype as much as anyone else… worshipping the gods of Conspicuous Consumption.

Now, I'm not a religious person, but I do believe in some higher, universal power, and I've grown to appreciate many of the practical aspects of the religions I've studied. Interestingly enough, almost every religious philosophy encourages and respects some form of good personal hygiene. The five faiths of Islam, Christianity, Judaism, Buddhism, and Hinduism all have age-old parables that speak of the spiritual importance of bathing and cleansing, to remove dirt as well as sin.

Muslims, Hindus, and Buddhists ritualistically wash before prayer. The symbolism of cleanliness of the body is a prerequisite of cleanliness of the soul. The Old Testament refers to Moses and Aaron washing their hands and feet to cleanse themselves of impurity. The New Testament's references to Holy Baptism represent a cleansing of the soul, and foot washing signifies humility and dedicated service to others.

In Buddhism, faith lies not in idealism or materialism, but in the reality of the here and now. Cleaning the body is akin to purifying the brain. To mindfully perform one's daily ablutions—washing, scrubbing, tweezing, trimming, and rinsing—is seen as an essential part of one's religious practice. Mindfulness in one's daily routine (whether cleaning one's home or one's body) can lead to a more meaningful, or even transcendental, human existence.

In many eastern philosophies, the universe is controlled by the interaction of the elements, which—when paired with the duality of the Yin and the Yang—create contrast, tension, conflict, and balance. Much like the five elements in Chinese medicine (wood, fire, earth, metal, water) and the five elements in Asian cooking (sour, bitter, sweet, spicy, salty), the five essential elements in *Clean Body* function according to a similar philosophy. All of the *Clean Body* elements are equally important and depend on one another for marvelous chains of reaction and interaction. It is the union, blending, and balancing of these elements that, I hope, will make for you and your family a mindful, integrated Zen-Cleansing experience.

The five pure elements used in *Clean Body* are:

Baking Soda
Lemon
Olive Oil
Salt
White Vinegar

Each of the components has its own task—singularly and in tandem with the others. None of the five are new-fangled or unusual, and they've been safely used for centuries. I'll bet that you already have all of them in your pantry. Now it's time to repurpose and rededicate them for a wonderful, healthy, non-toxic, and eco-friendly beauty regimen.

So, while "new and improved" ultra-fabulous but untested beauty products are being piled high on store shelves, humble Baking Soda, Lemon, Olive Oil, Salt and White Vinegar await you, ready to prove themselves as excellent, beneficial alternatives. They are absolutely reliable, and they hurt nothing—after all, you probably eat all five on a daily basis. Plus, they really clean.

Clean Body basics will necessitate some simple storage that you'll need to supply. Plastic tubs, spray bottles, and covered glass jars that you probably already have—quick, dive into that recycling bin!—will work fine. Zen-Cleansing is nothing fancy. Just make sure the containers you recycle are absolutely clean. Remember, the packaging from all the commercial products we throw away will probably outlast us and generations to come. By doing the simple, mindful act of recycling what's already in your home, just imagine all of the plastic and glass that will no longer need to be manufactured, and how much less will end up in landfills or recycling centers across the country. It's a small act, but multiplied by millions of households, it can have real impact!

Each of us can be a powerful catalyst for change by putting our consumer energy where our hearts are. Just remember, if we don't buy their products, they won't make them. It's really that simple. And until they can prove to us that their commercial personal hygiene products are safe, sane, pure, and ethically tested, *and* until they are transparent about what's in them, we can use these old-fashioned, tried-and-true alternatives that our grandparents and probably their grandparents used for generations and generations.

Clean Body is not just about bodily hygiene; it's a philosophy, a mindset, and an alternative to mass consumerism. By combining this with other attempts to protect ourselves, loved ones, families, friends, and beloved pets, we can reclaim the environment, force big business to have a conscience, and restore our little part of the world to the Eden it once was.

In Zen teaching, our mind and the universe are one, and our thoughts and actions meld into realities. In Zen-Cleansing, the goal is for us to come face-to-face with ourselves during any chore we take on. Through feeling, looking, hearing, tasting, or touching, we can achieve this.

With all that in mind, let's try something different. We all need to bathe, wash our hair, moisturize our dry skin, brush our teeth,

25

and groom ourselves, so why not try cleaning with the safest ingredients we can get our hands on? Follow the simple and nontoxic recipes I've provided in this book, and take pride in the fact that you can mindfully and safely clean yourself, your babies, your beloved or betrothed—and pass these tips on to anyone else who looks like he or she could use a good scrubbing, too.

THE INGREDIENTS

THE INGREDIENTS

BAKING SODA

Fresh from its familiar, iconic compact carton, the white, soft, and dusty-dry gems of baking soda shimmer like Caribbean sands. Its potential barely tapped, an open box of baking soda is probably already hiding in your refrigerator, forgotten behind the onions and oranges, anchovies, apples, and other endless edibles—effectively absorbing any disagreeable odors. *Clean Body* will change all that.

From the ashes of burnt corncobs, pioneers made early baking sodas named saleratus, trona, or nitre. Found on the shelves of frontier homes as well as in the traveling Medicine Man's bag of talismans and herbs, it was prescribed as a cure for everything from asthma to eczema and bellyaches. It transformed animal fat into treatments for chapped skin and did double duty to clean floors, scrub pots, and shine shoes.

Hygiene with baking soda, however, goes back a lot further than the Wild, Wild West—all the way back to Biblical times. "For though thou wash with nitre, and take thee much soap, yet thine iniquity is marked before me, saith the Lord God" (Jeremiah 2:22). In ancient Egypt, when used to mummify the remains of great pharaohs, not only did baking soda clean the body, but preserve it as well. Established in the beds of Egyptian lakes, the crystals form when water in the heated desert climate evaporates. Traded for thousands of years, Egyptian writings as old as the reign of Ramses III refer to these deposits.

Sprinkled, scattered, spread, or strewn, kept in your closet, kitty litter, crisper, or carport, baking soda—under any name—is totally safe yet powerful enough to preserve the dead. (Kids, do not try this at home!) Today, its strength can be used to sweeten, clean, and freshen your home and body. Baking soda is the most effective and probably most often used ingredient of the five basic cleansing agents. But this is more than just a forgotten freshener for your fridge, a way to pickle a pharaoh, or a tub scrubber. *Clean Body* will show you how to use those powdery white flakes to transform yourself into a "Baking Soda Beauty."

LEMON

Strong, sharp, acidic, and citrus-sassy, the golden-hued, egg-shaped lemon—whether picked ripe from the tree or found in the produce section of your supermarket—offers sun-ripened effervescence. Grown among sharp thorns and twigs, oblong leaves, and fragrant reddish buds that blossom into white and lavender flowers, the lemon fruit is oval and aromatic. Its memorable scent is produced by oil glands dotting the tough exterior of rind, under which lie the tender, juicy segments. For some, the thought of a lemon makes their mouths water.

The eight to ten perfect sections hidden within the leathery exterior offer up what was once prized by sultans, gifted by kings, and traded across the continents by sailors, pirates, and smugglers. Although the lemon's origin is unknown, it is believed to have been cultivated in ancient Mesopotamia and Egypt, and it is rumored that Christopher Columbus carried its seeds in his vest pockets. Today the tart and succulent fruit is grown in Italy, Spain, Greece, Turkey, Cyprus, Lebanon, South Africa, Australia, the Philippines, and here in the States.

Not all that long ago, the now humble lemon was highly coveted by adventurous seafarers and pillaged by plunderers. In the process, the vitamin-C-rich crop made its way from continent to continent, used by sailors as a preventative for scurvy. Nowadays most of us get our "C" from a balanced diet or by taking supplements, but back then, lemons were precious and necessary cargo.

With names like Armstrong, Bearss, Berna, Eureka, Femminello Ovale, Genoa, Harvey, Interdonato, Lisbon, Meyer, Monachello, Nepali Oblong, Nepali Round, Perrine, Ponderosa, Rosenberger, Rough Lemon, Santa Teresa, Sweet Lemon, and Villafranca, the common lemon may not be just "oh-so-common" after all. Each variety varies slightly in color, texture, shape, flavor and scent. But whether you choose the exotic or the mundane variety, any lemon you can get your hands on will certainly do the trick as far as your "clean body" is concerned.

Lemons aren't just for fish and tea anymore, as you'll soon see! *Clean Body* will show you how to re-purpose this magical fruit from a mere tangy garnée to a bunch of beauty recipes. Whether sliced, halved, or whole, you can achieve the softest of hands and feet, apply salon-like hair streaks, make a fabulous facial astringent and acne deterrent, prevent or eliminate dandruff as well as bad breath, and even quickly deep condition your hair. Who-da-thunk-it?

A bowl of a dozen placed casually out in the open, another bunch tossed into your crisper, and a small custard dish filled with cut pieces stashed in your refrigerator door will make living with the most perishable of the five ingredients all the easier.

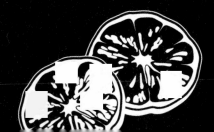
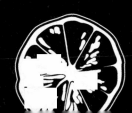

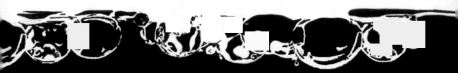

OLIVE OIL

Whether pale yellow, olive green, or honey-amber, olive oil is remarkably versatile. Like honey, it requires no refrigeration, making it easy to store and use. And whether cold-pressed, virgin, or extra-virgin, this traditional, luxurious oil has long served as much more than the main ingredient in the perfect vinaigrette. As you'll soon discover, it is also a nourishing beauty aid.

Available just about everywhere—from gourmet shops to the local bodega—olive oil is considered a basic household staple, and it has been used for a variety of non-food purposes throughout the centuries. Mohammed used its richness to anoint himself and the heads of his disciples, and it is often used for baptism in the Christian faith. This yummy unguent was also used to bless early rulers as well as winning athletes. Olympic champions are still crowned with wreaths of olive leaves, a tradition established at the first ancient Greek games,

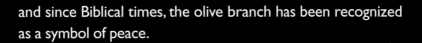

and since Biblical times, the olive branch has been recognized as a symbol of peace.

Used in the burial process in ancient Egypt, it was believed that the fruit, branches, leaves, and oil of the olive tree, when included in the departed's sarcophagus, would ensure a safe and pleasant passage to the underworld by protecting the souls of the dead from evil spirits.

Clean Body will teach you how olive oil can protect you from other "evils"—dry skin, wrinkles, chapped lips, and so on. From now on, when it comes to smoothing and maintaining your skin and hair, you'll be a champion in the "Beauty Olympics" by anointing yourself with these amazingly effective and chemical-free olive oil treatments.

SALT

Lustrous, brilliantly white, and crystalline, salt is one of the most plentiful and useful minerals on Earth. We enhance our culinary creations with it, melt icy sidewalks with it, and many cultures have created parables about it. Planets in outer space are filled with ginormous bubbling, molten oceans of it, while here on Mother Earth we race cars on Great Plains of it, buoyantly swim in tropical turquoise-colored oceans of it, and even "take the cure" in it. Stored in shakers displayed on dining tables or found next to stovetops in heaping bowls, the coarse, granular, or powdery pale mineral stands ready to offer the handy pinch to almost every sweet or savory culinary concoction. And while you'll still shake it over your eggs, now *Clean Body* will have you scrubbing your legs (and other body parts) with it!

Listed on the periodic table of elements—and known to us also as iodized, sea, bay, kosher, canning, pickling, or rock salt—sodium chloride occurs naturally in the soil and water. Salt is the fourth most abundant element on Earth and, like baking soda, was used to preserve the remains of the ancient pharaohs.

No less than thirty references to salt are made in the Bible. Lot's wife was transformed into a bloodless pillar of the stuff when, even though she was warned not to, she just *had* to turn to see the fall of Gomorra.

Roman soldiers of antiquity were often paid in salt, and this was called their salarium, from which our word "salary" is derived. It was said a soldier was "worth his salt," a term still used today to describe a worthy person. Once paid with salt, a soldier could use it as money in exchange for other goods.

Superstition has it that if spilled, you should toss some salt over your left shoulder to ward off bad luck. Not that I believe it, but ..ya' know, it can't hurt. Don't waste too much of it, though— it's far too useful! Salt actually is worth its weight in salt! It's not just practical in the kitchen or for homemade housecleaning projects; the plentiful common table salt stands alone in its beauty applications. As you'll see, it's an extraordinary exfoliator, super sterilizer, dynamic disinfectant, and an ample antiseptic. Forget about old Ruth in the Bible—with these Zen-Cleansing salt recipes you'll become a "pillar of prettiness." Let's exalt salt

WHITE VINEGAR

Vinegar, from the French for "sour wine," is produced from assorted fruits, berries, melons, coconut, honey, beer, maple syrup, potatoes, beets, malt, grains, and whey. But the production, in essence, remains unaffected—no matter what its original form. First is the fermentation of sugar to alcohol, and then the fermentation of alcohol to vinegar. Simply put: fermented fruit? Voilà! Acetic acid is born.

Sharp, sour, and biting—to most of us, the tang of vinegar always remains the same. But the flavor of one type of vinegar to another is very different. There's wine vinegar, rice vinegar, apple cider vinegar, tarragon vinegar, balsamic vinegar, and any number of other exotic blends.

But for "bodily" purposes, look for that familiar yet forgotten bottle of clear, distilled "white" vinegar that's probably lurking in your pantry, hidden behind the condensed milk, cans of coffee, spring-form pans, and cookbooks. This multipurpose elixir can linger eternally—refrigerated or not—making it easy to store and use. The pungent and sparklingly piquant, crystal-clear liquid is versatile, gastronomically and otherwise. Vinegar is not only a flavor enhancer, but also a literary and Biblical metaphor, an age-old cure-all, and a homespun cleaner. Vinegar has become a fabled figure of speech used to describe feisty folks, been referenced in the Chinese allegory of the Vinegar Tasters—tasting sour to Confucius, bitter to the Buddha, and sweet to Lao-tzu— and been used to shame Jesus (in Psalm 69), in each case causing generations to ponder its allegorical, legendary meanings.

The ancients stumbled upon the versatility of vinegar probably 10,000 years ago. The Greeks used it as medicine and flavored their meals with it. The Romans drank it as a beverage. Cleopatra dissolved pearls in it to prove she could devour a fortune in a single meal. Biblical references show how it was used for its soothing and healing properties, and as recently as World War I, vinegar was still being used to treat wounds in the battlefields.

Susan B. Anthony was considered the "vinegar" of the women's suffrage movement. By being aggressive, breezy, ebullient, frisky, spunky, and full of vitality, she displayed the classic traits of being full of "piss and vinegar," a phrase made popular by John Steinbeck in his novel, *The Grapes of Wrath*.

It is said, "You catch more flies with honey than you do with vinegar," implying the virtues of sweetness over bitterness. But in the case of *Clean Body*, it is precisely the acidic virtues of white vinegar that make it such a sweet beautifying treasure. Just like olive oil, store plenty in a tightly sealed container and keep it close at hand because many *Clean Body* recipes rely on this deliciously "bitter" potion.

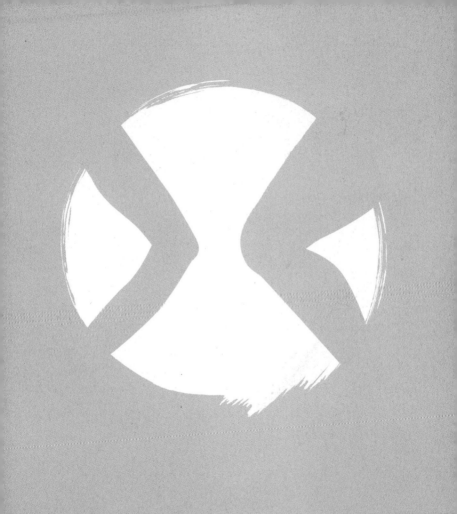

ELBOWS & KNEES

ELBOWS AND KNEES

"Now my soul hath elbow-room."
~WILLIAM SHAKESPEARE, *KING JOHN*

Unable to swing a tennis racket or to even brush their own astonishingly blonde hair, Barbie and Ken first hit the toy market without so much as a bendable knee or elbow. These mechanical "disabilities" ironically restricted their ability to drive, even though they had a car specifically designed for them. Ken couldn't get into the traditional position to propose, and neither one of them could climb the stairs in their "Dream House" without awkward hopping. Heck, Barbie didn't even have a bendable elbow from which to swing her mod purse!

Just imagine a world where our major joints didn't bend. The Statue of Liberty couldn't clutch her big green torch and tablets, *The Thinker* couldn't support his chin while he pondered, and poor old *Mona Lisa* would be surly from standing rather than comfortably sitting with her arms elegantly crossed.

An elegant dining experience wouldn't be nearly the same—you'd have to always stand, and someone else would have to feed you! The elbow and knee aren't given much thought, but they are clearly very significant pieces of the human anatomy.

And for reasons apparent only to Miss Manners, it's never appropriate to put your elbows on the table while dining. (C'mon, you do it too!) In fact, the typical start to my day includes propping up my still half-asleep head on one hand, with an elbow serving as a support on the counter, and holding my cup of coffee with the other. Often I'm either leaning on my elbows while I read the morning paper, or more likely blankly staring out into the garden, daydreaming about what I need to do that day, or—dare I say it—pretending to listen with rapt attention to my partner, who is a morning person whereas I am so definitely not!

Yet the clearly important elbow and the other major joint, the knee, are usually given short shrift when it comes to our beauty regime. Often somewhat dry and numb to the touch, knees and elbows are meant to offer flexibility, dexterity, and locomotion. These all-important joints are covered with thin yet highly resilient and hyper-flexible skin that sees a lot of action within the course of the average day. Used to push through a crowded subway car in true New York style, elbows also offer us an amazing spot to place a hand while walking with a friend or someone special. And the ability to crawl on all fours is not only the first mode of personal mobility for an infant; it allows us to look for lost keys under the sofa, dust bunnies under the bed, or that renegade bar of soap. In our lifetimes, we have all found ourselves crawling around on our elbows and knees at one time or another.

Brilliant in their design, our elbow and knee joints allow us a graceful range of motion with which to move elegantly and freely through the world—well, perhaps not so elegantly in every case (you've never seen me on a dance floor). Our major joints allow us to be very bendable and limber, giving us the physical options to be ever-changing and adaptable. But they also bear the brunt of physical wear, and because of this, they require special care and attention. Knees and elbows need a mindful *Clean Body* working over to keep them in tip-top shape.

BAKING SODA

- To **smooth elbows** and **knees**, make a paste of baking soda with just a few drops of water. Work it into your elbows and knees, rinse well, and then follow with just a dribble of olive oil on the same area. Rub the oil in. You'll notice a huge difference even after the first time you try this.

- Okay, you've been gardening. I'll bet you're in need of an elbows and knees **deep cleaning**. Place a bit of baking soda into a moist washcloth and give it a good scrubbing to reveal the clean skin hiding out just beneath the grime.

SALT

• To exfoliate, lightly massage salt into your knees or elbows. Take a warm damp cloth, sprinkle salt onto the folds, and gently rub over the rough areas in small circular motions for just a few minutes. An **elbow** or **knee exfoliate** reveals fresh, healthy skin just below the calluses. Remember to rinse very well with warm water and finish by patting it dry with a fresh towel.

LEMON

• Hack a lemon in two. (Now, didn't that feel good?) Cupping a lemon half in your hand, rub your elbows into the juiciest, fleshiest part of the fruit—first one, then the other—giving equal attention to each for about five minutes. Oh no, you're not done yet. Have a seat, 'cause you're gonna do the same thing to your knees. The acid in the lemon will "tenderize" those much-used joints (think ceviche!), soften pesky **elbow** and **knee**

calluses, and even reduce dark patches. If you can, just leave the juice where you applied it for about fifteen to twenty minutes, then shower it off to discover softer, paler skin. Pat dry.

• No need to suffer with **discolored elbows** and **knees**. These darkened patches are easily lightened with a repetition of lemon compresses and hot water. Rub with freshly sliced lemon (remember to use the juicy side!), and just let it sit there for about fifteen minutes. Find something to do—make a call, file your nails…then, using a hot, wet towel, scrub like the dickens to slowly remove the discolored skin. (This will take several attempts, if your knees look anything like mine did.) Be patient: they didn't get that way overnight, and they won't clear up overnight either.

WHITE VINEGAR

- Pour a quarter of a cup of white vinegar and one and a half cups of warm water onto a soft compress, then apply to your aching, tender, or **sore elbows** or **knees** for roughly ten minutes, two to three times a day (or as needed).

OLIVE OIL

- You know it's gonna dribble from the bottle anyway, so do yourself a favor: catch those drips and rub them into where they will do the most good. Your supple, **soft elbows** and **knees** will thank you for it later.

FACE

FACE

"Plain as the nose on a man's face."
~CERVANTES, *DON QUIXOTE*

In the morning, I wake up face-to-face with someone I love. It makes me smile. Maybe you should try it too—smiling, that is.

Try this: For a moment, actually feel where your lips are when you smile. Does the top lip touch the lower lip? Or are your lips arched in an upward curve, teeth peeking through? Every smile is unique, yet our ability to smile in response to a pleasant thought is a quite remarkable universality.

Recalling someone or something, a special place, a pleasant memory of a moment past or of one about to occur brings a sincere smile to your lips. How wonderful it is that a pleasing thought–sweet, endearing, or just plain funny—can give us the strength to move mountains by merely turning up the corners of our mouth and wrinkling up the corners of our eyes. Crows feet and that map of well earned "character lines"—if you're my age and not using Botox—turn upward into the sides of your face, temples, and hairline to halo each of your eyes. Your body produces pleasant warmth 'til each of your cheeks blush pink, if not red. A hearty smile grows 'til it fills your entire face and overflows and spills to your ears and to your tongue and expands in your mouth and then deeper inward or perhaps straightaway out in the form of a sigh, a giggle, or a deep belly laugh.

Now I'm no Cary Grant, Rock Hudson, and certainly not Marilyn Monroe, or even Brad Pitt for that matter, but my face—just like yours—distinguishes me from everyone else. My extra long forehead (I'm bald!), stubbly chin (I hate to shave), blue eyes, pinkish white skin, long, thin nose, Frans Hals–like pinchable reddish cheeks, mouth, and lips are mine and mine alone, separating me from all others—including my twin sister, Margaret, with whom I share several facial features. Through them I display my joy, desire, worry, angst, anger, pain, and excitement. My facial features allow me to communicate with the world without ever speaking a single word. The endless variations on the theme of a face—eyes, nose, mouth, cheeks, chin, ears, forehead, hair, etc.—make each of us unique. But what we all share is the universality of a smile, a frown, and a million other subtle and not-so-subtle ways to communicate nonverbally with just the slightest lift of an eyebrow, squint of an eye, flare of a nostril, and so on.

Regardless of who we are or where we live, our faces are exposed for the entire world to see. The simple routines in *Clean Body* are an owner's guide to, literally, "saving face." The practice of daily, gentle cleansing and mindfulness in our actions allows us to put our best face forward. To achieve this, there are just five basic rules to consider:

1. Use plenty of water.

2. Don't wash it too often.

3. Never scrub it too hard.

4. Remember: always, always, always rinse well.

5. Everyone around you is stuck looking at it, so treat your face with care.

BAKING SODA

• In a gentle, circular motion, apply this homemade **facial scrub**: a brew of three parts baking soda to one part water. Rub the scrub in gentle circles from your forehead to your jawline to you chin, taking your time as you go. Rinse super well to reveal a clean, fresh-scrubbed mug. No need to towel yourself; just let your skin air-dry.

SALT

• Put the warmest water you can tolerate into a large bowl or sink. Standing directly over the steaming basin, throw a clean towel over your head to capture the swirling vapors. In minutes you'll unlock the pores—those thousands of holes in your hide. Remove the towel, stir one-fourth cup of salt into the warm water, and splatter it onto your fine features. In the event that you have razor burn, small cuts from shaving, irritations, or just plain old pimple-problems, salt is a swell **facial antiseptic**.

Follow immediately with a dash of fresh and frosty H_2O to re-close your pores, and pat dry.

- Just a tiny bit of the finest-grained table salt makes a **facial exfoliate and disinfectant** for your skin. Pour a pile into your palms and massage it into your face with warm water. (Don't get crazy here—it's your face, not a fry-pan.) Work gently in round motions for no longer than a minute, douse with clean water, and dry thoroughly.

- **Pimple, blemish, or zit, the common white head** need not ruin your plans for an evening out on the town. Join one-half teaspoon of salt to one cup of lukewarm water. Once dissolved, with a tissue or cotton ball, apply, dip, and reapply this tonic to the offender several times to help diminish the overall inflammation.

LEMON

• Apply lemon juice with a cotton ball to maintain your stunning skin. As a **facial astringent**, it removes excess oil and kills creepy bacteria. Pat some onto your face every morning. Leave it alone to do its thing for about ten minutes or so, and then rinse it off with tepid water followed by your favorite moisturizer. By just wiping some fresh lemon juice onto your face daily, you'll be amazed at how soft your skin will become. Make sure to avoid your eyes.

WHITE VINEGAR

• For **facial acne**, apply vinegar nightly by dabbing full strength with a cotton ball. Before you know it, your reddened skin will vanish to reveal a healthy, glowing version of itself in just a few short weeks.

• Oh, that super-shiny, slippery, **oily face**! A greasy slick from ear to ear, or just in spots, can be eliminated by mixing one tablespoon of white vinegar with one cup of water and rinsing daily to face a beautiful new you.

• To prevent rashes and irritations, use white vinegar full strength as a brilliant **aftershave**. It's not cologne, mind you, but it will comfort your tender skin.

• A homemade **facial toner**, made of 50/50 water to white vinegar, will tighten and firm your flexible face.

OLIVE OIL

• Just a drop or two of the purest unadulterated olive oil dribbled directly into the palm of your hand will have you saying bye-bye to your favorite commercial **facial moisturizer**. Apply to an already clean and wet face, and allow it to air dry. Easy does it, though—less is certainly best here.

It's hard to keep a straight face if you're not.

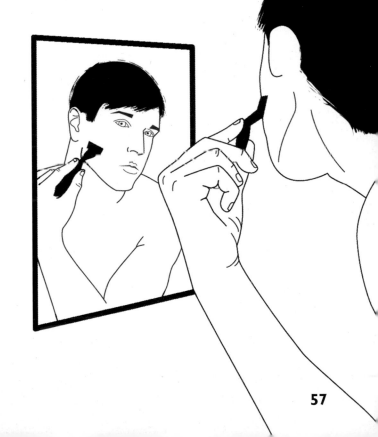

• Olive oil used full strength makes a marvelous **makeup remover**. Fill a cotton ball and wipe away. Hey, it worked for Cleopatra… It'll work for you, too!

RECIPES

• Forget about the expensive junk. Treat yourself with a **moisturizing "spa" facial scrub** at home using raw ingredients you've already got on hand. Start by getting your face completely wet with warm water. With your fingers and palms, liberally work a small palm-sized puddle of olive oil into your face. Once well applied, add about a half-teaspoon of fine salt to your palms and lightly scrub your face 'til it feels cleansed. The salt works great as an exfoliator, and the olive oil helps keep your face youthful and dewy soft. Remove any remains with a warm, wet cloth. (To complete that spa experience, follow by slowly sipping a cup of herbal tea, taking a three-hour nap, and visualizing yourself buying an oceanfront condo in Spain! Mmmmm…)

FEET

FEET

"A lamp unto my feet and a light unto my path."
~PSALM 119:105

From prehistoric times to the not-very-distant past, walking meant trodding the earth, often in sandals, crude shoes or boots made from animal pelts, and often even barefoot. Arid meandering through desert sands, dry, clay dust or clinging, wet mud, accompanied by annoyingly painful rocks and pebbles, frostbite-inducing snow and ice, and the occasional splinter from the rare wooden walkway defined the daily activity of getting from one place to another on foot. Talk about "my aching feet!" Remember, McAdams only invented macadamized roads within the past 150 years. Up till then, it was all dirt, dirt, dirt, mud, and, did I mention, dirt?

And for various civilizations and religious groups, the exposure of feet to the elements made the act of foot washing–either with water or oil or sand—quite an important and sacred matter. Spiritually, the act of foot washing is a repeated theme in most religious texts, and is used to illustrate a loving, compassionate act symbolizing humility and selfless giving. For instance, the New Testament tells the story of Mary Magdalene bathing Christ's feet with her tears and drying them with her hair. And in many other religions, it is the sacrifice as well as the blessing of the godhead to wash the feet of the masses—including those whom the rest of society has shunned, such as the poorest of the poor, the homeless, the ill, lepers, etc. Feet also play an important role in fairy tales like Cinderella, and are used in home truths like, "walk a mile in my shoes." Tender tootsies have been bound or even tortured into stilettoed symbols of feminine beauty, and are often fetishized as sexual objects.

In our modern world, hidden beneath socks and shoes are our heels, insteps, arches, ankles, soles, and toes, giving us remarkable stability and mobility—even when teetering perilously in Manolo Blahniks. Our feet come "upholstered" in assorted skin types— everything from the leathery, sun-baked, tough, and calloused to the pampered, pedicured, and porcelain smooth. In a typical lifetime, our feet will make over one hundred million steps. The amazing feats of feet allow us to stand, walk, run, dance, jump, drive, ski, and swim. They're the part of our body that regularly connects us with the planet, and, conversely, they are the part of our anatomy that allows us to leap from it as well. They meet the floor first when we start each day and are the last body part under the covers when it's all over.

My feet are small-ish…Hey, I know what you're thinking, but that's an old wives' tale! I'm over six feet tall, but with my size-nine shoe, I am often teased that I don't have a very firm footing. Large or small, doughy and round or slender and thin, I'd venture no two people's feet are quite alike. And while in some cultures it's completely inappropriate to show a bare foot, in others it's just as wrong not to. But whether they are exposed or not, dressed up or down, bound up or ornately decorated with henna, toe rings, nail polish, and ankle bracelets, I think we can all agree that the best way to put your best foot forward is to make sure it's clean.

Clean Body feet are washed daily, dried completely, and, depending on your personal circumstances, powdered or moisturized. Stop your "dogs from barking"; the following recipes will help you keep your feet happy!

Sell your soul and lose more than your feet.

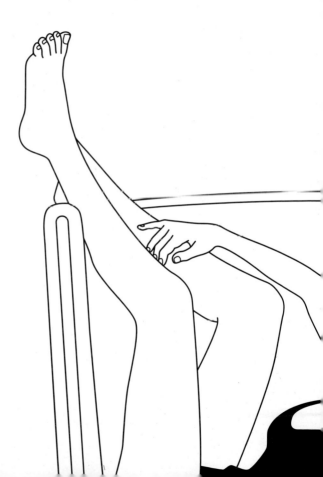

BAKING SODA

- Sprinkle four tablespoons of baking soda to one quart of warm water. This **foot soak** for frazzled feet takes only ten minutes and leaves your tootsies fabulously squishy-soft and smooth.

- If you have **stinky feet** . . . Perhaps the best way to fix that is to wash them more frequently. Additionally, changing to fresh socks or stockings daily plus a dusting of baking soda as a low-cost **foot deodorant** might just be a step in the right direction. If you're not wearing socks or hose, try sprinkling the baking soda directly into your shoes to eliminate odor and moisture.

SALT

- For **athlete's foot**, steep your feet in warm, salted water (one teaspoon of salt per cup of water) for five to ten minutes every day. The salt kills the fungus and reduces perspiration. When finished, dry each little piggy thoroughly.

LEMON

- When you're dead on your feet and your **burning soles** and **heels** need extinguishing, soak your barking, biting dogs in hot water for ten to fifteen minutes and follow by massaging each foot with juice from a sliced lemon. Leave the juice on for a few minutes, then rinse your feet with cool water and dry them thoroughly. You should feel a dramatic cooling.

• Kiss those cranky corns goodbye! For natural **corn removal**, every night place a slice of luscious lemon onto your calloused area (the fresh and pulpy side of the lemon face-down). Wrap it with cotton gauze to keep it from migrating in the night. The offender will turn tender and soon disappear.

WHITE VINEGAR

• Wouldn't it be nice if getting **athlete's foot** meant you were actually an athlete? Make foot fungus a thing of the past by wiping your peds with vinegar before you crawl into the sack. (Sure, it might sting a bit, but get over it—remember, you're an athlete. Toughen up!) Repeat morning and night until the infection has cleared.

OLIVE OIL

- Infinitely better than baby oil, the tiniest bit of olive oil will soften your feet from your ankles down. Regularly paired with clean, white cotton socks overnight, expect this **foot moisturizer** to leave your tender tootsies sexy, soft, and supple.

RECIPES

- For smooth, sweet feet, combine one cup of lemon juice, two tablespoons olive oil, and enough warm water to fill a foot basin. Soak your peds for fifteen minutes, then rinse them under warm water and pat dry. Once a week is all you'll need to have noticeably **soft and smooth feet**.

• Resuscitate your feet with a refreshing homemade lemon juice and olive oil treatment. Red, rough, and rugged feet will find cool comfort with a lemon juice **foot massage**. Cut a lemon in half, and rub the pulp side all over each foot, getting into every crack and crevice and all around each toe, ankle, and heel. Rinse your "lemoned" feet under warm running water and finish off with a few drops of moisturizing olive oil rubbed onto your refreshed tootsies.

• A once-a-week **foot tonic** in ankle-deep bath water with a "shot in the arm" of one-half cup of vinegar and two table-spoons of salt will leave your tired dogs feeling revitalized and rejuvenated. Just do it and don't ask why…you'll thank me later. You'll probably even want to do it more often!

HAIR

HAIR

"Even a single hair casts its shadow."
~PUBLILIUS SYRUS, *MAXIM 228*, 42 BCE

We all have hair—more or less. Some of us even have it where we don't want it! Fine, medium, coarse, wiry, thin, thinning, or thick; straight, curly, wavy, or kinky; normal, oily, or dry; blond, brunette, red, salt-and-pepper, silver, gray, or a whole host of colors in between: henna, apricot, chestnut, sable, cinnamon, fawn, ecru, winter-white, or beige … light blonde, copper-brown, honey-red, ginger-twist, sun-kissed, winter-wheat, or ash—no matter, it's all hair. And maybe the color's naturally yours (yeah, right!), or maybe you've just paid a small fortune for it. The possibilities are as limitless as the hairs on your head—all 120,000 of them (for those who still have a full head of it.)

I actually have a lot of nerve writing about hair. Perhaps someone more "follicly gifted" than me—with hair resembling the luxurious tresses of Lady Godiva, the voluminous strands of Rapunzel, or the virile mane of Sampson—would best write this section. Don't get me wrong, I have hair…but, unfortunately, most of it is at home clogging my drain.

I'm not totally bald. I have an unusually huge forehead with a healthy ring of blond mixed with salt-and-pepper stubble. Barbershops and, for that matter, shampoo are no longer part of my grooming routine. Instead, I hang my head over the bathroom sink every week and buzz my male-patterned coiffure down to a permanent five o'clock shadow. It's amazing how my three hairs look just like four when I'm done! Lucky for me, my lack of hair has grown on me. No wigs or rugs here. I personally wouldn't think of wearing a toupee or growing a comb-over—I'm bald and proud!

Daily care with wholesome products can help keep your hair—if you've got it—strong and strikingly beautiful. When you're shopping for your product of choice, keep this in mind: if you can't pronounce the ingredients, they're probably not that great for you. Once you've made your selection and finally commence the act of shampooing, remember to massage your scalp slowly but thoroughly with your fingertips, vigorously stimulating the circulation of blood. Feel the tension release while your digits activate your locks right down to the roots. Even us baldies can benefit from this! Then, rinse thoroughly. And while every commercially bottled shampoo says, "Wash, rinse, and repeat," ask yourself, "Says who?" The "repeat" is less designed to properly clean your hair than it is to sell more shampoo! Only "repeat" if you're in the mood, or if your hair is so filthy that you think you need it. Let's not split hairs: it's good health and mindful grooming that make for beautiful locks, not standing in the shower, endlessly "washing, rinsing, and repeating." In fact, you can "repeat" yourself into a head of dried out frizz if you're not careful.

So, whether your tresses are presented as a comb-over, corn-rows, crew-cut, flat-top, pigtails, or pompadour, here are some *Clean Body* suggestions for their continued health, beauty, manageability, and all-around well-being.

BAKING SODA

- For a simple **shampoo replacement**, combine one table-spoon of baking soda with two tablespoons of water. It won't look anything like the shampoo you're accustomed to; it's really more of a **shampoo-paste**. So for now, just pretend it's shampoo, okay? (And there aren't going to be those moun-tains of crazy bubbles either. They only occur because of the chemicals put in commercial shampoo to make it lather up.) Work the paste through your hair and rinse thoroughly. You can expect clean and remarkably shiny hair.

- To revive dreary and deadly dull hair, combine one quarter of a cup of warm water with the sufficient amount of baking soda to make a watery-wet **hair-clarifying paste** (think pancake-batter consistency). Just dump it into your wet tresses. Comb, rub, kneed, massage, and moosh it all around. Do what ever it is that you need to do to make this act more exciting for yourself, and when you're utterly bored of the experience, rinse thoroughly to reveal a spectacular, shimmering mane.

• No more excuses for that dirty, oily hair. **Dry shampoo** to the rescue! Dust the smallest amount of baking soda into your dry hair and put your busy little digits to work by massaging it down to your roots. The baking soda will zap the oil and capture most of the dirt. Shake your "do" to remove the excess powder, pull a comb through your hair, and you'll look like you really had the time to groom.

SALT

• My only recommendation is to avoid any recommendations regarding the use of **salt on your hair**. Never do it! It gobbles up natural oils and can transform your otherwise luxurious locks into a snarl of straw in a nanosecond. Steer clear!

LEMON

• For a pristine spring, shine, and sheen, mix the juice of one lemon with one cup warm water and apply to your otherwise dull "do." Take a powder for about fifteen minutes and let your homespun **citrus quaff-conditioner** sit pretty, then rinse thoroughly. This will add a new bright-bounce and glow.

• For the cost of a lemon, create your own subtle **salon streaks and heavenly highlights.** Apply the juice of an entire lemon to your dry, untreated, newly shampooed, clean hair. Really get in there, with this stuff covering the shaft from root to tip, and then simply abandon it there to dry totally. (Don't rinse it, don't comb it, don't even drag a towel over it—*just leave it alone already.* Ignore it. Pretend it's your Amex bill or the guy you had drinks with last weekend.) Allow to dry completely. Repeat if desired for even more depth and shine. Note: This is **not** recommended for chemically treated hair.

WHITE VINEGAR

- Yet another thing to make your hair shiny? Sure…why not. If the lemon thing wasn't enough for you, or you're just a shine junkie, rub your scalp and massage your hair each evening with a solution of 50/50 vinegar and water. This **hair-product-residue remover** leaves behind the glistening, polished hair you've always dreamed of.

OLIVE OIL

- For healthy locks with unbeatable shine, this delightful **moisturizing hair treatment** helps speed restoration to your worn and tattered split ends. But, like a Ronco product, it doesn't just stop there. It does so much more. It also nurses the scalp back to health, eliminating those nasty flakes and making your locks silky-smooth—and shiny, to boot! Knead a few tablespoons of olive oil into your scalp and hair. Swathe your moisture-soaked curls with a plastic bag and abandon it there for thirty minutes.

Bald men have silent explosions, not bangs.

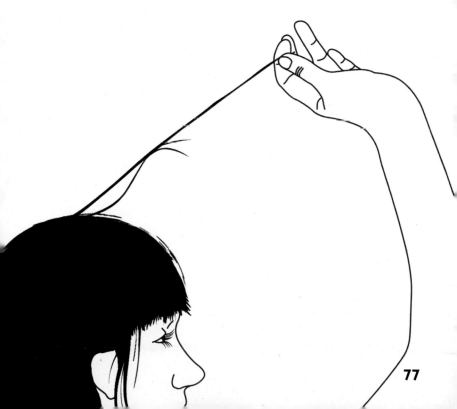

Snooze, toss back a latté…whatever. Shampoo as usual to reveal a refurbished mane that even Fabio would envy.

• Nobody likes **kinky hair,** even on a good day. But here's a solution that will **rid-the-frizz**. Put the smallest dribbly drop of olive oil into your palms and fingers. Massage it into your hands and then drag your fingers through your already dry hair. Style as usual.

RECIPES

• Why not **make your own shampoo**? At least for once you'll be able to pronounce all of the ingredients. Begin by tossing one ounce of olive oil, an egg (yes, a raw egg, —eeesch!), a single tablespoon of lemon juice, and a half-teaspoon of vinegar into your kitchen blender. (But be sure to rinse that remaining margarita mix out of it first!) Give the shampoo ingredients a spin, and then lather it in. Use this mixture right away: this one's got a super short shelf life because of the egg. You're certain to love it.

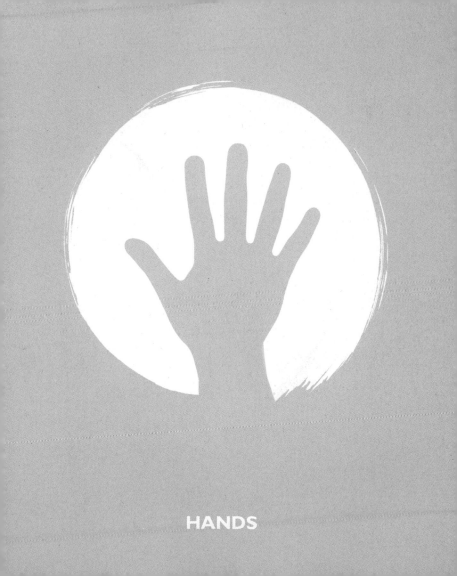

HANDS

HANDS

"For Satan finds some mischief still for idle hands to do."
~ISAAC WATTS

My hands are my vehicle. Neither decorated with a Hindu's henna or an heirloom from Harry Winston, they create the chicken potpies, paintings, and the wistful words that I'm known for. They repaint the walls of our home at every whim. They sew on buttons, make beds, pet our dog, fold and sort laundry, drive screws, pull weeds, and arrange flowers. Besides that, they also help me communicate by punctuating my words and the air around me with abstract yet necessary movements.

Digits, opposable thumbs, palms, nails, and wrists—whether you compose proclamations, harvest produce, prepare meals, play pianos, or put out fires, your hands are the most dexterous appendage you have. What's more, hands are in large part what separate us from other life forms (that, and our ability to accessorize, of course!). Intimately associated with this body part is our sense of touch, through which we are able to assemble feedback and react physically to the tactile world. We make manifest our dreams with our hands and, likewise, leave behind our fingerprints on the world. For good or for bad, hands have "had a hand in" raising up civilizations and then extinguishing them over and over again.

So don't become a modern-day Pontius Pilate or Lady Macbeth by letting your dirty digits get out of hand. *Clean Body* hand-washing is easy to learn, and is probably the most important way to prevent the spread of germs and colds to others around us. Try the following, and it's "out, damned spot!"

1. Fill the plugged up sink always using warm water.

2. Add soap and lather up your palms, digits and the backs of our hands for at least twenty seconds—about the time it takes to sing "Twinkle, Twinkle, Little Star" (in your head, please!).

3. Use a nailbrush to scrub away caked-on dirt or paint and to clean the grime from under your fingernails.

4. Rinse well with fresh running warm water.

5. Dry thoroughly.

HANDS

BAKING SODA

• Gardening can be treacherous to your talons. After an afternoon of crawling around in the dirt pulling weeds, transplanting
plants, or burying bulbs, my paws are always a raw, rugged, filthy
mess. (I guess I could use gardening gloves, but that would spoil
the fun!) I get my hands spanking clean with my favorite **hand
cleaner**: baking soda, some warm water, and a nailbrush. Pour
a one-inch pile of baking soda (about a rounded tablespoon)
into your lightly dampened hands and scrub the daylights out
of your cuticles, fingers, palms, and wrists. You'll still have hands
that look like they've been doing hard work, but at least there
won't be any remains of the day's dirt.

• Whether you're after pretty palms or handsome hands, a weekly baking soda **hand soak** is a momentary calm in the storm of everyday life. Begin by stirring two tablespoons of baking soda into a basin of comfortably warm water. Plunge those babies right in and leave them there to pickle and prune for the next thirty luxurious minutes—yes, a full half hour! Leaving you incapable of multitasking is the hidden strategy behind this soak: you'll find some rest and relaxation, not to mention soft and sexy hands. Without rinsing, next drip the smallest bit of olive oil onto to your still warm and wet hands and proceed to let them air-dry.

SALT

• To eliminate calluses, soften unsightly rough patches, and offer yourself an amazing **hand exfoliation**, place a hearty tablespoon of table salt into your olive oil–soaked palms. Starting lightly and building gradually to a more aggressive massage, rub the salt into your hands, wrists, and elbows to reveal glowingly fresh skin. Rinse with warm water and pat dry.

LEMON

• Lemon juice is an amazing tenderizer for crusty knuckles, arid elbows, parched palms, and flaky fingers. Cut a lemon in half and scrub the sloppy, moist, juicy-fruity part into your skin. Let it do its hocus-pocus by allowing it to sit for about five minutes. Rinse thoroughly. Meant not only as a **hand softener**, it also leaves them smelling, well, just like lemons!

*Is it possible to know palm reading
like the back of your hand?*

WHITE VINEGAR

• Stinky hands are acceptable only if you're an offshore fisherman lost at sea somewhere. To the rest of the civilized world, there's no excuse. Intended to banish potent garlic or fiendishly foul fish from your fingers, this swell **hand deodorizer** works to eliminate the stench: simply rinse liberally with white vinegar.

OLIVE OIL

• Buttery-soft hands are a symbol of wealth and leisure. Yours can be that way, too, even if you're the handmaiden—and not the mistress—of the house. Just slop some olive oil on your paws before bedtime. (Cotton or rubber gloves will keep the oil off the sheets and on your hands, where it belongs.) Come daybreak, your **moisturized hands**—wrists to pinkies—will be silky and soft.

• If "desperately dry, dull, desiccated, and dehydrated" describes your personality, you've got problems that this book can't address! If it describes your cuticles, however, relax. We're here together to fix all that. Parched cuticles needn't be gnawed, chewed, or scraped off. Just a drop of olive oil massaged into your fingertips daily as a **cuticle conditioner** will keep them pliable and pretty.

• Crispy claws? Flimsy fingernails? Toughen your manicure by soaking your nails in warm olive oil. This five-minute **nail hardener** is all it takes. Truly!

RECIPES

- If your hands are reddened, rough, and raw…maybe you work part-time as a lumberjack. Regardless of whether you harvest timber for a living, perhaps your sore, tired hands could use some TLC with a **moisturizing hand treatment**. Begin by rinsing them with pure lemon juice, rubbing it into the most felonious areas. Next, rinse under warm running water, and follow by massaging them with warm olive oil. (Lemon juice and olive oil make a great salad dressing, too!)

MOUTH

MOUTH

"Nature has given us two ears but only one mouth."
~BENJAMIN DISRAELI, EARL OF BEACONSFIELD

Mine is a busy little place. It houses my tongue, gums, tonsils, lips, teeth, and that little wiggly thing way back there called the epiglottis. Collectively, all of these features allow me the ability to yawn, sing, eat, cry, drink, speak, smile, frown, kiss, hiss, and sneer.

I'm told I have a big mouth because I talk way too much and, yes, I even laugh at my own jokes—often more than others do! I sometimes sing when I think nobody's listening (even though I swear I have a great voice), but my favorite pastime with what the English so lovingly call my "cake hole" is eating. However, because we put any number of delicious tasty treats into our yappers over the course of any given day, it's the part of our bodies in need of most frequent cleaning. Maybe the cat's got your tongue, or you just put your foot in your mouth—either could leave you with a bad taste, though not in the same way an onion bagel can. So, let me teach you the *Clean Body* way to keep your mouth fresh, clean—and infinitely kissable!

BAKING SODA

- Just one teaspoon of baking soda in half a glass of water makes a pretty terrific **mouthwash**. Stir it up, swoosh it around in your mouth for a good twenty seconds, spit it out, and then douse your mouth with fresh, cold water. This is not a mere minty camouflage; the offending aromas will actually be a thing of the past!

- Sparkly white teeth are an asset, and a clean mouth is the only way to start the day fresh. We've all had a morning when, to our horror, that tube of **toothpaste** is squeezed and pinched into a figure eight, and there isn't even the tiniest bit loitering in the underside of the cap. Try using baking soda to help keep your ivories clean. Shake some baking soda into the flat of your hand, give your brush a dip and revive your pearly whites. Brush, brush, brush, spit, and rinse.

Sometimes your foot can be found in your mouth,
next to the skin of your teeth.

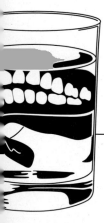

SALT

• Just a pinch of salt into a glass of water creates an excellent substitute for the more classy antiseptic and posh herbal **oral rinse** sold over the counter. Gargle away! It'll also help alleviate a sore throat and soothe painful gums.

LEMON

• You just had the tuna wrap laden with shallots, paired with an enormous garlic pickle. It's a good guess that your breath is bound to offend someone back at the office. Try chewing on a fresh lemon wedge as a midday **breath freshener**. Swish the juice around to help remove that ghastly breath.

WHITE VINEGAR

• Dip your dentures in whole-strength white vinegar for about fifteen minutes to half an hour (or overnight, if you wish) and then give them a good brushing. As a **denture cleaner**, the vinegar will make them fresher and whiter than those dumb tablets in a box ever could.

OLIVE OIL

• There is nothing less appetizing than a beautiful face with angry, split, and peeling chapped lips. To relieve and repair the damage from the wind, cold, and sun, dab olive oil directly onto your parched puckerer for instant **chapped lip relief**.

PRIVATES

PRIVATES

"As soon as you deal with [sex] explicitly, you have to choose between the language of the nursery, the gutter and the anatomy class."
~C. S. LEWIS

You'd think that speaking about this stuff would be easy, especially by someone like me. I've proven to myself and others that I can write about anything: Groundhog Day, Christmas, Elvis Presley's birthday. And sure, I'm an adult (well…chronologically speaking, at least), but when I began thinking about writing this book, I decided that I wasn't going to write about anything that would make me uneasy. So I went ahead and wrote a manuscript, managing to skate my way around anything that has anything to do with anyone's "rudey bits." And when it was all said and done, anyone who was anyone said to me, "What? No rudey bits?" Thus, I figured I'd appease the "few" individuals who actually have them by writing a chapter entirely committed to cleaning one's "secret garden."

The bare truth often has consequences.

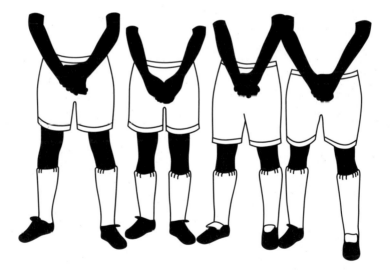

Our "tender vittles," male and female, are our private organs specifically created for reproduction or just plain pleasure (among other things). We most commonly keep them quietly hidden away beneath clothing to protect them from the hazards of everyday activities (swinging baseball bats, slamming doors, hot stoves, opening filing cabinets…ouch!) as well as the scorching rays of daylight—not to mention public decency laws.

But because they are so reclusive, these delicate tissues, which are often sensitive to soaps, deodorizers, and detergents, need special care and attention.

(Remember: If you have any questions or feel uneasy about trying any of the following recommendations, please consult your doctor.)

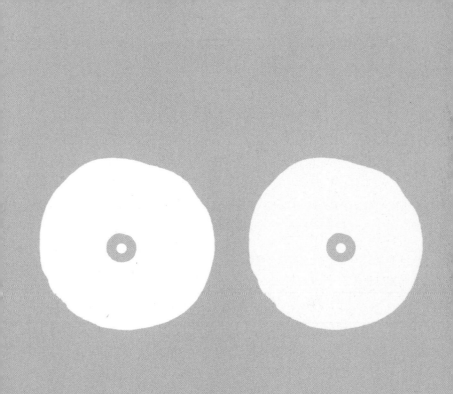

PRIVATES *for* **HER**

TA-TAS

PRIVATES *for* HER

TA-TAS

"I think it's about time we voted for senators with breasts. After all, we've been voting for boobs long enough."
~CLAIRE SARGENT

"Thelma & Louise," "knockers," "melons," or perhaps you simply call them breasts—the glandular, fatty, and fibrous tissue found directly over a females pecs are what makes them so completely squashy-spongy-supple-silky and pleasantly soft.

Although breasts aren't involved in the "Dirty Deed" (well, not directly, anyhow) and don't facilitate creation, they're important because they not only look swell in a bikini, fill out the bustier of a strapless evening gown, offer delightful eye-catching curves ("the bigger the better, the tighter the sweater"), but also because, regardless of their size, they very effectively feed newborns.

(Note: All women over twenty should give themselves monthly breast self-exams. Please check out the Susan G. Komen for the Cure site at www.komen.org for free, potentially life-saving information!)

BAKING SODA

- The entire breast and nipple may be cleaned with baking soda and water after breastfeeding to keep **duct openings** free and clear.

SALT

- Every woman should wash her breasts daily. A **weekly soak** in a warm bath mixed with a half cup of salt makes it difficult for organisms to grow on them, thereby keeping the "girls" healthy and happy.

LEMON

- A bath with fresh lemon slices reduces **skin exhaustion, inflammation, and irritation** that may result from the tight elastic and scratchy in-seams of brassieres and other "restrictive" garments (or going braless!).

WHITE VINEGAR

- After breast feedings, a mother's **nipples** can be rinsed with a solution of one cup water plus one tablespoon white vinegar to keep them soft, healthy, and ready for baby's next meal.

OLIVE OIL

- **Stretch marks**, either from exercise, puberty, yo-yo weight loss, or pregnancy, may be alleviated by treatments of olive oil. Go ahead after your shower, while your skin is still a bit damp—a dribble will go a long way. Air dry so your skin can absorb the oil.

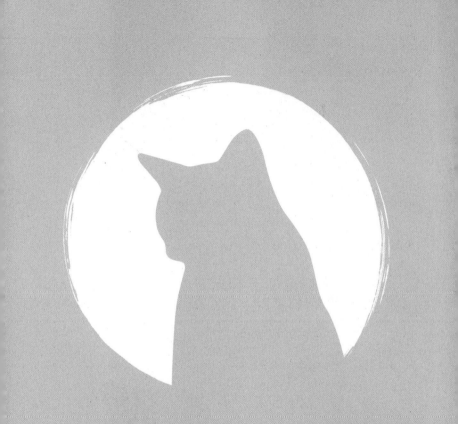

PRIVATES *for* **HER**
FERTILE DELTA

FERTILE DELTA

Charlotte: "Oh my god! Vagina weights!"
Samantha: "Honey, my vagina waits for no man."
~SEX AND THE CITY

Many consider women's genitalia to be unmentionable—apparently even Oprah. The "va-jay-jay" is a remarkably flexible yet versatile part of the female anatomy. Lots of folks (including myself), however, feel some awkwardness when using the word "vagina." Luckily, playwright Eve Ensler came along and gave it a monologue! Offered pseudonyms such as "honey pot," "easy bake oven," and "Oval Office," and averaging a depth of between three to six inches, the vagina is elastic, muscular, effectively spectacular when it comes to the "fun stuff," and nothing short of miraculous when it comes to childbirth.

Whether you're a nymphomaniac searching for her G-spot, or a nun ignoring hers, the female orgasm is actually a powerful painkiller. *Sooooooo*… "Honey, I have a headache," is, in fact, a lousy excuse not to be doin' the "horizontal mambo."

BAKING SODA

• Add one cup of baking soda to one quart of warm filtered water for an effective **douche**. Allowing the mixture ten minutes to completely dissolve, apply with a clean, handheld bulb-douche or douche/enema bag nozzle.

SALT

• Dissolve one-quarter cup of salt in your bath. Salt water promotes healing and may **prevent infections**.

LEMON

• Because of its antiseptic properties, a solution of water and lemon juice can be used for **itchiness**.

WHITE VINEGAR

• In a time-honored tradition, before commercial perfumed douches were marketed (ask your grandmother), the vinegar douche was the original **vaginal cleanser** of choice. Add two tablespoons of white vinegar to one cup of warm filtered water for a gentle, natural douche. Again, as with the baking soda douche above, apply with a clean, handheld bulb-douche or douche/enema bag nozzle.

OLIVE OIL

• Toss the whipped cream and chocolate sauce out of the shopping cart, because anything "food"-related—including olive oil—down there is just a plain ol' bad idea.

PRIVATES *for* **HIM**
WEDDING TACKLE

WEDDING TACKLE

"Alas, the penis is such a ridiculous petitioner.
It is so unreliable, though everything depends on it—
the world is balanced on it like a ball on a seal's nose."
~WILLIAM GASS

Slightly south of the equator of every man, you'll find what some laughingly call the "fun gun," "Kojak," "baloney pony," "tallywhacker," "tool," "trouser snake," "wood," or "John Thomas."

With history replete with leaders who have often seemingly thought with their manhood and not their minds, this exclusively external male reproductive appendage has often been influential in guiding past and present world events. Although the rhinoceros has a "codger" of approximately two and a half feet long, and understanding that most men are notorious liars in that department—whether it's a grower, a shower, or somewhere in the middle—we male mammals can at least breathe easy in the knowledge that our "equipment" is much larger than any other primate's.

Each culture and every religion has its own quirks: medical procedure or not, circumcision is no day at the races, but it is, unfortunately, permanent. (Nothing like petunias that grow back in the spring.) But whether it be "snipped" or left "natural" ("cut" or "uncut," "crewneck" or "turtleneck"), the average adult male's "hidden treasure" becomes aroused every time he dreams, and may still be potent well into his seventies. By keeping your "hardware" clean, you, too, can expect to keep the old "kick stand" in working order for years to come.

(Oh, and just so ya know, studies have proven that smoking can shorten your "gadget"—just another reason for kicking *that* nasty habit.)

Is it cocky to say that size doesn't matter?

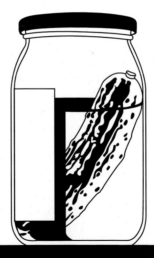

BAKING SODA

- A dusting of baking soda after a bath or shower will keep your "fruit basket" **dry and fresh**.

SALT

- Every male should wash his "unit" at least once a day. Men with foreskins especially need to attend to this, and should pull their "hoodie" back to assure cleanliness. In addition, however, a simple warm **weekly bath** with a half cup of salt makes it difficult for organisms to grow, thereby keeping you healthy and clean.

- After washing, pat your "Johnson" down and let it air dry.

LEMON

- Your "organ" is highly sensitive. Applying lemon juice on your "21st digit" might cause minor burns. Avoid it: you'll be showing your "javelin" some respect.

WHITE VINEGAR

- Wash your "Easy Rider" frequently with white vinegar *highly* diluted in water. For any kind of **genital irritation**, vinegar baths are spectacular. Remember: never apply straight vinegar to your "gherkin"—you're not pickling it, you're just cleaning it.

OLIVE OIL

- Massaging your entire body (yes, *everything*) lightly with olive oil will greatly enhance skin tone and **smoothness**. Apply it while you're still damp from a bath or shower, and let yourself air dry so your skin absorbs the oil.

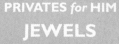

PRIVATES *for* **HIM**
JEWELS

JEWELS

"No matter how much you feed a wolf,
an elephant still has bigger balls."
~RUSSIAN SAYING

"Doo-dads," "coin purse," "giblets"—if you're a healthy male, good guess is you have two testicles, paired side by side, neatly packed away in your scrotum, handsomely located outside of your body, suspended underneath your "Action Jackson."

Sensitive to heat and cold, the "cojones" relax and tighten in response to changes in temperature, your choice of underwear, and during sex.

(Note: All men over the age of fourteen should self-examine their "business" once a month. Visit the Testicular Cancer Resource Center site at tcrc.acor.org for easy-to-follow, illustrated directions.)

BAKING SODA

• When your "gooseberries" are reddened, a full cup of baking soda in the bath helps with **rashes and itching**.

SALT

• In the event of an **inflammation**, a splash of salt water will do the trick. Or you may soak in a tub filled with warm water and one cup of salt.

LEMON

• Because of its **antiseptic** properties, diluted lemon juice may also relieve itchiness, but never use the lemon full strength— the acid could cause more irritation

WHITE VINEGAR

• Take a long, hot bath with one cup of white vinegar added to relieve a case of **jock itch**—the "twins" will thank you.

OLIVE OIL

• The occasional light dressing of olive oil will keep your "tea bags" **soft and supple**.

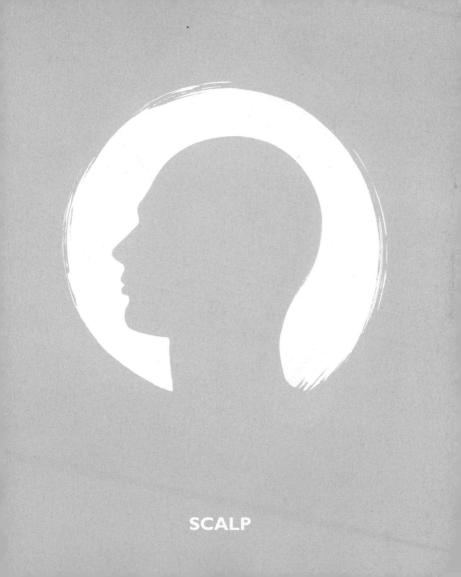

SCALP

SCALP

"Thou anointest my head with oil; my cup runneth over.
Surely goodness and mercy shall follow me all the days of my life."
~PSALM 23

The scalp is not just a habitat to heaps of hair (or not so many heaps, if you're "follicly challenged" like me!). Rather, according to disciples of yoga, it's where you connect with the highest branch of who you are, your crown *chakra*. Directly translated, that means "a thousand petals of a lotus," and it's where we tune into and surrender to divine consciousness, join with immeasurable energies, understand the unfamiliar, and feel the transcendental meanings of life, oneness, and joy.

Located just below where your proverbial light bulb goes "on," your scalp starts where your hairline begins and ends in the folds of the nape of your neck. It's from whence our tresses grow… or used to grow. Soft and thin-skinned, the scalp easily chills and warms, and next to our face and hands it is the part of the body that has almost continual exposure to the elements. Our dome

118

is where we lose our body heat the quickest, and conveniently, it's also where we can wear a hat to make sure that doesn't happen too often.

The scalp is also the part of our body that's closest to the sun—that is, of course, for those of us who haven't buried our heads in the sand! But regardless of which direction our scalps are pointed, there are Zen-Cleansing tips to help you mindfully care for this often unconsidered and highly neglected body part.

BAKING SODA

• Day after day, you squeeze out gobs of gooey gels and moun-
tains of messy mousse to get that "do" of yours to do what
it does. (This applies to men, too, so listen up!) After hours
of preparation, a fine mist of finishing spray allows you to
greet the world looking kind of windswept and "fresh." (Who
knew "natural" could be so much work?) Make some time to
de-glop your hair by starting each day with a **scalp-clarifying
rinse** of baking soda and warm water to remove any of those
dry and crusty, torturous chemical remains on your crown.

SALT

• Salt is nice on eggs. Some folks even like it on their cantaloupe.
It's super effective on an icy sidewalk and swell at keeping your
water pipes from freezing in the dead of winter. But unless you
really want your bangs to look like a whiskbroom, just know
that salt in your hair and on your scalp is a bad idea.

LEMON

- Dandruff isn't glamorous. So, rather than toss out your favorite little black dress or your cherished dark suit, give this a try. Begin by hacking a fresh lemon in two and squeezing half of the lemon directly into your hair for a wonderful **dandruff treatment**. Schmoosh it around, and do your best to make certain it comes in contact with your entire scalp. Wash your hair with either your favorite shampoo or one of the recipes you'll find in this book, and then rinse well with warm water. Do this every other day or until the dandruff disappears.

- Just because I don't have hair doesn't mean I can't have an **itchy scalp**. The juice of an entire lemon applied to the "old chrome dome" does wonders. (It's great for those "afflicted" with hair, too!) Massage it in before you shower, and let it just do its thing for about five minutes or so. (Shave your legs or your chin, trim your sideburns, pluck your ears…find something to do. As we all know, beauty is a mean mistress!) When done, hop into the shower and rinse.

WHITE VINEGAR

• Vinegar works well on that uncomfortable dryness that often leads to **pesky dandruff**. Rub white vinegar into your hair and scalp for just five short minutes before you shampoo. Wash and rinse as usual.

OLIVE OIL

• Believe it or not, olive oil smothers **lice**—they just hate it. Rub enough to thoroughly coat each strand—the amount here will differ from person to person—working it in from your scalp all the way to the tips of each hair. Let the oil sit for at least thirty minutes—even longer is better here. (That is, if you don't have any better plans. But where do you want to go with lice, anyway?) Then, wash the oil out completely. You might need

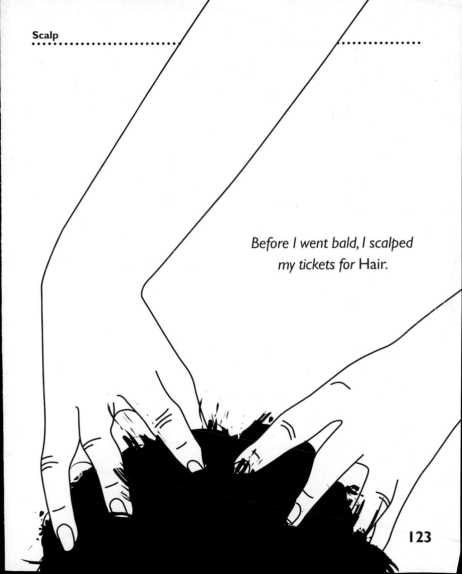

*Before I went bald, I scalped
my tickets for* Hair.

to shampoo several times to eliminate the olive oil from your hair and scalp. If you don't have lice, do this weekly as a **deep-conditioning scalp treatment** and effective defense against dry scalp and hair.

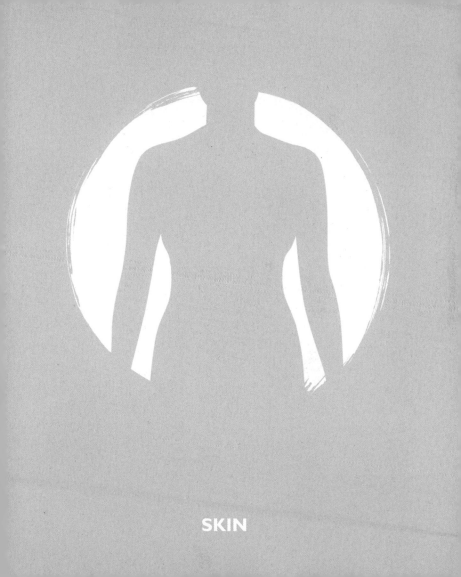

SKIN

SKIN

"It is not the color of the skin that makes the man or the woman, but the principle formed in the soul."

~MARIA STEWART

Like many people, I love to be touched, and likewise I love to touch in return. I often touch a new acquaintance's arm while I shake his or her hand for the first time. I place my hand in the niche of a friend's elbow while we walk. Without words, I welcome others by offering a welcome and friendly touch.

Our skin automatically responds to the world around us, whether we realize it or not. We sense the warmth of our environment and respond to heat by cooling ourselves with moisture—perspiration pools in the small of our back and our armpits, and it peppers our chest, legs, forehead, and upper lip with droplets of salty water. We also warm ourselves with the subtle vibrations of shivering or by getting goose bumps when exposed to the cold.

We all vary so much from one another, but especially when it comes to the color and texture of our skin. Personally, I am the

*You don't need to be in the flesh
to get under somebody's skin.*

quintessential pale-boy, thanks to my Dutch heritage. I practically disappear when it snows! If unprotected, I sunburn easily, painfully, and quickly, and it takes me a full two weeks smothered in SPF 45 to even get the semblance of a tan. My partner, on the other hand, is olive-complexioned, and goes from a wintry "green" to bronze on the first day of a vacation in the sun.

Whether you are among the palest of the pale, pink, salmon, yellow, olive, red, tan, mocha, mahogany, or ebony; whether you are porcelain-like, freckled, wrinkled, velvety, rough as sandpaper, or smooth as a baby's bottom; remember that the skin is the body's largest organ. It's what holds you together, so it would be wise to take are of it. Mindful *Clean Body* care will protect you, no matter what skin you are in. Be kind to your hide: clean skin is healthy skin.

1. Bathe daily.

2. Use plenty of water.

3. Lather up with the gentlest of cleansers.

4. Don't scrub too hard, but hard enough.

5. Always rinse well.

6. Then, rinse some more!

BAKING SODA

- Give yourself the most fantastic face and **all-over body scrub** with baking soda. (Really. This is one of my *most* favorite tips!) Your skin will glow with a newfound polish. To eliminate those dead skin cells, leaving your skin soft, tender, and smooth, create a three-to-one paste of baking soda and H_2O. Massage it gently all over your face and body. Follow by rinsing well with warm water and allowing your skin to air dry. Do it every day, and watch the transformation. (They even did this in Biblical times, only they called it *niter*, instead. A rose by any other name…)

- Tossing half a cup of baking soda into your bathwater is an amazing **skin softener**, leaving your hide feeling downright sexy. Pick a night, fill the tub with the hottest water you can tolerate, light some candles, put on some soothing music, and see what happens.

SALT

- In a heated skillet, prepare a **poultice** of coarse salt. Place the warmed salt into a paper bag and apply it directly to your affected, achy areas.

LEMON

- For **itchy skin relief**, apply whole-strength lemon juice to the dry and scratchy areas. Just chop that little guy in half and give it a squish. Leave the lemon juice there 'til it dries, and then rinse thoroughly.

- Squeeze some lemon juice into a clean bowl or jar to create a homemade, lemony **astringent**. Fill a cotton ball and pat it on any oily patch every morning. Ten minutes is all it takes. Rinse it all off, and wash with warm water. Keep any remaining lemon juice in the refrigerator for the next application.

- Apply lemon juice directly to **acne**-afflicted skin. It does wonders. Dab the acidic juice on the blemish, leave it to dry, and then rinse clean.

WHITE VINEGAR

- Whole-strength white vinegar spritzed onto a nasty **sunburn** will offer loads of relief. Begin by rinsing your skin in a tepid shower, lightly toweling yourself dry, and finish by spraying the vinegar wherever you need it. Reapply every other hour.

- Add one half cup of white vinegar to your bath water to relieve **head-to-toe itchiness**: This is another favorite of mine—soak in the hot vinegary water for fifteen to twenty minutes, and towel dry without rinsing.

• Apply a 50/50 combination of a white vinegar and water solution under your arms and any place else that produces "questionable" **body odor.**

OLIVE OIL

• Dry skin belongs on an iguana. Yours can be touchably yummy again with a spritz of olive oil mixed with water. Mix one-third olive oil to two-thirds water in a small, clean spray bottle to offer yourself an exhilarating after shower or bath **all-body moisturizing treatment**. Let it soak into your skin without towel drying.

• While running a hot bath, add about one teaspoon of olive oil beneath the tap. Rub the **bath oil–infused** waters into your face, body, and feet, and then soak for at least fifteen minutes.

RECIPES

- Mix together equal parts of extra virgin olive oil and salt to create a wonderful **skin softener**. Mix the two, so that the salt soaks up the olive oil, and then scrub your entire body, head to toe. Expect to be energized as well as exfoliated. Massage the mixture into your body and wash off thoroughly. You'd pay good money for this treatment if you were at a spa!

- Cut two lemons into super-skinny slivers. Dribble half a dozen drops of olive oil onto the citrus slices. Give it a toss, and finish with three cups of sea salt. Then, it's hands off while the concoction cures for at least five minutes. Add your **citrus derma-dip** to a hot and steamy bath. Lock the door, put on some soothing music, and submerge yourself into the citrus mix by loosening up and settling down for a long, luxurious, lazy soak. Reappear recharged and revived. You owe yourself this one!

- Liberate yourself of dead skin cells with this awesome **all-over exfoliator.** Blend three quarters of a cup of sea salt or coarse kosher salt, three tablespoons of baking soda, and one-quarter cup of olive oil in a bowl. Jump into a warm-to-hot shower, douse yourself down, dip a washcloth into the mixture, and scrub everything you can reach with the all-over exfoliator. Rinse well. Find your newly revealed, stunningly soft skin sparkling fresh and re-energized.

PAMPER YOUR SKIN NOW...

Sexy skin is as easy as doing nothing.

Ø Abuse.

Be gentle. Tender pats and soft strokes are the way-ta-go when cleaning, applying or removing makeup, shaving, or doing any of the bazillion things you might do to your skin over the course of a day.

Ø Arid air.

Pretend your skin is a houseplant. It, too, gets thirsty. If it looks and feels dry, it probably is. Treat it to a spritz or a generous splash of water regularly.

Ø Booze.

Alcohol will dry you out, period. Just a bit is fine, but any more than that and you'll be looking like a leather change purse before your time. Besides, a hangover is never pretty!

Ø Drugs.

Prescription medications will say whether or not to stay out of the sun, and whether or not they need to be taken with plenty of water. The other "funny" stuff messes with your mind and makes you dumb as topsoil. Use your judgment: if smashing skin is your goal, my good guess is that recreational drugs shouldn't be part of the program.

Ø Smog.

Pollution is hard to avoid. However, a regular rinsing with plain ol' water every once in a while during the day couldn't hurt.

Ø Smoking.

Bette Davis, Bogie, and even Lucy & Ricky sucked on idiot sticks. They didn't know better back then, but we do now. It'll mess up more than your pretty face. How about some chewing gum instead? Please, no gum snapping!

Ø Over-cleaning.

You've only got one "outfit" of skin this go-round. If you play your cards right, it should last about a hundred years. Treat it gently.

Ø Sunshine.

Daylight and sunbeams are pretty, but excessive sun exposure will mess with your skin. Use caution, listen to your instincts, and never go out without sunscreen.

Ø Yo-yoing.

Watching your waistline is important. But, come *on*…Find a weight and stay there. The ravages of weight loss and weight gain show because your skin is not a rubber band. Plump is prettier than stretch marks. Remember to eat lots of whole, unrefined grains, and drink plenty of fresh water, 'cause if the junk in the junk food doesn't come out one way, it will find a way out through your hide.

TUSH

TUSH

"On the loftiest throne in the world,
we are still sitting only on our own rump."
~MICHEL DE MONTAIGNE

Our glutes are the largest muscles in our lower backside, and these are what—along with plenty of fatty cushioning—makes it so round and shapely. Our tush's large size is one of the most characteristic features of the muscular system in humans.

It's our "bum" that allows us to sit upright, and it even supports us while we stand. Butt—pardon the pun—no matter how tough yours is, harsh soaps or wiping vigorously can chafe your skin, leaving you irritated and uncomfortable. Whatever you choose to name it—"derriere," "tuchas," or "buns"—hygiene is important for a healthy hiney. Daily gentle washing will keep yours clean.

BAKING SODA

• Your hiney will be shiny by scrubbing yours daily. Yours too can feel like a baby's bottom no matter what your age. Begin by massaging a three-to-one paste of baking soda and H_2O gently all over your cheeks (the ones *down there*). Follow by rinsing well with warm water and allowing your skin to air dry.

SALT

• Dissolve one-quarter cup of salt in your bath. Salt water promotes healing and may prevent **infections.**

LEMON

• Because of its antiseptic properties, a solution of water and lemon juice can be used for **itchiness**. And let's be honest, everyone has an itchy butt at some point in time.

WHITE VINEGAR

• Add one half cup of white vinegar to your bath water to relieve an **itchy booty**. Just soak in the hot, vinegary water for fifteen to twenty minutes, then towel dry without rinsing.

OLIVE OIL

• Massaging your tuchas lightly with olive oil will greatly enhance **skin tone and smoothness**. Apply it after a bath or shower, while you are still damp, and let your cheeks air dry so that the olive oil gets absorbed into your skin.

Cracking jokes leaves you the butt of them as well.

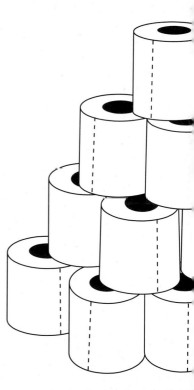

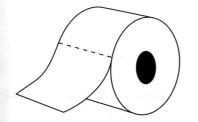

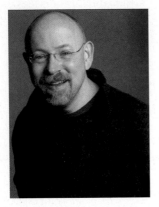

Author Michael DeJong is an environmentalist and eco-activist.
His blogs can be found at www.MyKindofClean.com

DeJong and Joost Elffers are generously donating all of the royalties from each of the books in the Clean Series to the OneCleanWorld Foundation, a philanthropic, not-for-profit organization that supports environmental projects worldwide with grants, technical assistance and/or micro-financing. For more information about the foundation, visit www.onecleanworld.org

To contact Michael DeJong, email him at Michael@MyKindofClean.com